For Rissa,

without whom this book would never have been written,
or even thought of for that matter.

Dedicated to all humans, and a dog named Jack.

Foreword

I became interested in health and wellness while working at UNC as a research programmer in nutrition and epidemiology. I decided to take a health and wellness course to learn more about food and how it helps (or harms) the brain/body. I fell in love with the course and in my free time starting reading research-based books (and articles). Being the nerdy person that I am, not only did I highlight and underline while reading, but I also decided to write those ah-ha passages in longhand. This was nothing more than my way of trying to remember and it was something fun to do with my spare time. After talking with my sister one day about some of my discoveries she said, "You should write all this down, maybe write a book with all the highlights so people like me don't have to read all those boring books." That's a much-condensed version of our conversation but you get the point. I had already started typing some of my notes as an attempt to solidify the findings in my brain. It wasn't a big leap to then put these together into short readable books. I hope my nerdy love of reading research-based books will help others who, like me, are trying to improve their lives a little each day. I know it will at least save you countless hours of reading. I hope you take away a nugget or two that will make your life healthier and therefore happier. It's a proven fact that healthier people are happier. I don't know who proved that, but let's get healthier people!

This book is just one chapter. It's designed that way. You only have to read one chapter and you can brag that you read an entire book. Doesn't that feel wonderful? Perhaps this book will be broken into sub-parts, perhaps not. I haven't decided yet. I'm just planning to type here till my little heart is content and stop somewhere before 100 pages. I read somewhere (although I don't remember where at the moment) that the adult attention span is about 20 minutes, on average. Most can drift for a brief moment and go for another 20 minutes of focus, again and again. I do not have that ability. I have the attention span of a flea, or perhaps more accurately, a fruit fly. I'm one of those (un)lucky people who at times drift off; literally nothing going on in the brain. I know it looks crazy to others when they see this happen to me. My niece saw it firsthand just this past weekend and I thought she might have me committed. I'm not even sure what happens. I was never tested. For goodness's sake, I was born in 1969 in the rural South. We didn't test kids back then. If a kid did something weird, they got sent outside to 'play'. I'm outdoorsy. Enough about that. I want you to know one other thing about me. I am NOT an expert on any one of these topics. Oh, and don't be confused, just because I work in research, I am not the researcher on any of the findings that I'm about to share with you. I am just a regular nobody sharing some nuggets of information that have made my life healthier and happier. I don't claim that any of this is really even accurate. You know how research goes, one day you can eat eggs and then next, you betta not. Cook it in margarine, no cook it in butter! Who knows what's right? Only math and logic have absolutes, science is constantly 'in progress'. All the research in the world just leads to the most wildly accepted theory. So, just read the book and take from it what you will; what fits for you. Do your own personal research. How your body responds to food is unique to you. Yes, we have things in common, but we are also quite different, and you need to figure out for yourself what works and doesn't work for you. That's part of the fun of life, finding what works for you and ditching what doesn't. In the back of this book, you will find Rae's Recipes. And trust me, you're gonna wanna try 'em all. Mainly, I ended this way because I have no idea how to end a book and 'Recipes' seemed like a good way to end a book titled The Body on Food. With each recipe is a few pages of writing space to evaluate each recipe and how you feel after following that recipe. You're welcome.

This page is intentionally left blank
(In case your mind has drifted, and you need to jot down a reminder to
get avocados at the grocery store later today).

Chapter 1: The Body on Food

Since this book is the body on food, I thought it would be good to explain what happens when we eat. For starters, our body triggers feelings of hunger when we get low on readily available energy. Because food is fuel, our body sends panic signals!!! "FEED ME! FEED ME, NOW, dang it!" What's going on here? We are wired to survive, and our body knows this instinctively, so when we get low on fuel (could be any nutrient or mineral that we need) our body sends up a red flag. The red flag has a name: ghrelin. I like this name, I'm gonna name my next grouchy cat Ghrelin. Doesn't this name look like something that we should all be afraid of? ('Don't get them wet!') In actuality, it's just a hormone. Yep, a hormone, that's right, like estrogen or testosterone, except Ghrelin's job is to let us know when we need fuel. Ghrelin, lovingly referred to as the hunger hormone, is produced mainly by the stomach, but small amounts can be found in the small intestine, pancreas, and the brain! See what I mean by RED FLAG? This stuff is everywhere, telling us that we are hungry and if ignored too long Ghrelin will become hangry. Because we are wired to survive, our body will send out ghrelin before we even use up all our fuel. So, when we're feeling hunger pangs, we still have fuel in the tank. What the heck? Speaking of fuel in the tank...our body will store roughly 1000 calories in the liver and muscles for immediate use. Anything over that will be delightfully delivered to our favored body fat storage sites for future famine use. Our body wants to avoid using fat storage for energy. Using fat storage is like telling our body that a famine has set in, or it's time for a hibernation or estivation. So, if you're trying to lose body fat right now, you are essentially in a battle with hunger and survival. Now you understand why intentional weight loss feels like that...because, it's actually true. What's worse is that we can, at times, still feel a craving even after eating. If what we eat isn't good for us, difficult to digest, or not what our body needs, this is our body telling us we need more nutrients. Hunger and craving can be triggered by a lack of nutrients, even just one, so we can feel physically full and hungry for something else at the same time. It's important to realize that not all vitamins and minerals have been categorized or discovered. We've even discovered some (B vitamins come to mind here) that are no longer considered essential or important enough to keep. (This explains the weird gappy numbering system for the B vitamins.) Pay attention to these odd cravings, they're telling us something. Next time you have a craving for something, ask yourself what is the predominant ingredient or spice or flavoring agent? Find the healthiest thing you can find with that ingredient and eat it. Satisfy the base craving as best you can. I wish someone would develop an App for this. So, when I'm craving something and I don't quite know what it is, I could lick my phone and Bing! I get a notification saying…"go eat some Brazil nuts, you're craving selenium right now."

Our brain wants easy fast energy even though what's best for it is slow steady energy. Brains can be like petulant spoiled children, wanting what they want and wanting it NOW! Truthfully, it's just trying to help us survive, in any way possible. Ever find yourself craving something sweet right after finishing a meal? Um, yeah, me too.

Here's a fun thing to try. Next time it happens to you, don't give in. See what your brain does. Does your craving drive you a bit nutso? Making you think about the sweet thing more than usual?

Note it in your personal research journal at the back of this book. The second time it happens, eat some fruit, berries perhaps. Pay attention to how this feels different than the time before. The third time, eat some cake. Note how that makes you feel afterward. We are made for eating natural sugars. The boost from natural sugar is the same as the boost from refined sugar, it's just that refined sugar is more immediate and therefore noticeable.

Once we've given in to Ghrelin and start to feed our hangry pie holes, we get a burst of dopamine (the "feel good" hormone), making us feel better than before we ate. "Yay, dopamine! Hello darling, I've missed you so much. Welcome back." But don't get too excited, it only lasts while we are feeling hunger. Eat slowly and enjoy your dopamine buzz because when eating at a normal speed leptin shows up in roughly 20 minutes and ruins the party. Leptin is the responsible older brother that tries to keep us in line. In other words, he's our satiation hormone that tells us when we're satisfied, which is actually a good thing! We all need a little responsibility in our lives, right? He lives in our fat storage sites, of all places! And can you believe that he gets his name from the Greek word leptos, which means…that's right, you guessed it… thin! Ridiculous. (Those responsible for the naming of body parts have a sick sense of humor.) Once Leptin appears, no more dopamine. Bye-bye feel-good neurotransmitter, hello responsible adult. Continuing to eat after this is just adding body fat for future famines. This seems like a good place to mention that there is such a thing as leptin resistance, a condition where leptin receptors are not functioning properly and when this is the case, dopamine will continue to flood the system. Sounds lovely on one hand, however, it's not. People who are stricken with this misfortune usually struggle with weight issues and the related diseases throughout their lives. I believe there are treatments available now, but I don't know enough about them to speak to those here so as my uncle Garland says, "I'm talking about something I don't know anything about, so I'll just shut up now."

HEY, I know something that might be fun…. Let's do a leptin test tonight. Try this…tonight at dinner eat very slowly, chew a lot before you swallow and take breaks, talk to your family, or if you're like me and don't live with a family, then talk to yourself. Time yourself and see how long it takes for your leptin to kick-in. Report the time to someone, anyone you can get to listen to you with your crazy notions about fun personal research projects. Good luck!

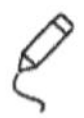 Write in your personal research journal how long it takes for your leptin to show up.

Let's back up, I got a little ahead of myself there. Once we start to fuel our bodies by consuming food, we chew, and our saliva covers the food and so begins the work of divine digestion. The more saliva that covers the food the better digestion will be. The more we chew food the more food is broken down and covered with saliva. This is good and really helps Mister Epi and Miss Uva. Mister Epi is the trapdoor for the throat that keeps us from sucking food into our trachea (otherwise known as windpipe) on most occasions, and Miss Uva is the little dangling fleshy thing in the back of our throat, which helps push food down the hatch rather than up our noses.

Stop now and go look at your uvula in the mirror. I'm fascinated by this little thing. Side story here, and perhaps explains my fascination. Sometime in the 1970s, my cousin Chris was running with an American flag in his mouth (true story) and fell, cutting his uvula, it's how I know the name of that weird thing! They bleed when they're cut. They also heal and grow back together. Neat little boogers. I wonder if his has a scar on it? I'll call him tonight. I would explain a little more about my cousin Chris, but I think this story says it all. In his defense he was probably 4 or 5 years old at the time, although I would NOT be surprised to see him doing this now in his 40s. And if you ask his sister Stefani, well, I'm sure she'd agree this is the only story you need to know about him. Now, back to the real story…Saliva has amylase which breaks down starches, and lingual lipase which breaks down fats; such helpful tools in the digestion process. Interesting sidenote – farmers carry a more active form of amylase than hunter/gatherers and are better at breaking down starches for absorption. I can't remember where I read this and who figured this out but, let's get to farming people!

Saliva is 99% water but has 1% enzymes, uric acid, electrolytes, mucus forming proteins & cholesterol. Yum! Ugh, again, who made up these words. Ooof! Regardless of how disgusting it sounds, their job is to begin the digestive process, which is a pretty crucial step, so let's just them do their jobs without judgment. Take your time, chew a lot, and cover that food in mucus forming proteins and uric acid, churn it all together into chyme and let Miss Uva keep it from going up our nose and Mister Epi keep us from chocking to death. For God's sake, don't be a speed eater. In fact, when you find yourself speed eating (and we all do it sometimes) ask yourself what unmet need or craving you might be trying to satisfy? I'll bet you'll find one. Just a hunch. After we've swallowed our food and it's finding its way down the hatch into the stomach...well, technically it's being pushed down there by a lot of muscle contractions which explains why we can swallow standing on our heads. Then, we get the next phase of digestion. Don't worry, I promise to stop this book before we talk about pooping. I read your mind, and I know you were thinking it, so I just wanted to get that on the table. No poop will be spoken of here.

The next phase in digestion is the stomach and its role. In the stomach, food finds its second level of destruction. This process actually begins when we smell food; remember the old Pavlov trick with pups? Entirely reflexive in its origin. When we smell something tasty, our vagal nerve is stimulated and that sends a message to start the gastric juices flowing. The stomach secretes acid and enzymes and churns food. It's basically a holding cell for the small intestine. When completely empty, the stomach is a little larger than your fist. However, it can stretch to about 12 inches by 6 inches and hold roughly a quart of solid food. Although the myth persists that thin people have smaller stomachs, it's not true. Most adults have similar sized stomachs, regardless of the size of the human. We do grow accustomed to how full we feel after meals and usually eat to that level of fullness at each meal (and sometimes for snacks). Thinner people may have a different 'thermometer' on what feels comfortable to them after eating. Can you feel your shirt right now?

Were you feeling it before I asked? I'm guessing that's a big N O. But, now that I bring it up, can you feel your shirt? YES, we all can feel our shirt and the first time our parents put one on us, we noticed it a lot! Maybe even cried a little getting it on. Or perhaps some smiled at the comfort of it, depending on your genetic predisposition. Our brains adjust to not noticing. This is a neat feature of our brains, it's part of evolution and survival. It helps us adapt and learn new tasks. Brain efficiency let's call it. We free up space in the brain when we don't have to notice things any longer. The brain actually competes for resources, meaning all parts of your brain can't fire at the same time. So, we have to not notice in order to learn something new. There would be no grad school education and research, if we had to always notice our shirts touching our skin. We would never have even learned to tie our shoes, we'd still be stuck trying to remember to poop on the toilet and not in our diaper. Ooops, I broke my promise. Sorry. Not noticing gives us the brain space to do things routinely so we can learn new things. Fullness works the same exact way. We develop a habit around how full we feel after eating and our brain logs that in as 'normal'. Anything less than that, feels like not enough. Anything more feels overfull. In the US, most of us have learned to overeat, to clean our plates, no matter how much was put on it. Over-eating is damaging. It makes us lethargic, tired, keeps us from moving as much as our body needs, spikes our blood sugar which leads to all sorts of problems we won't go into right now.

I see a Body on Sugar book coming soon. The good news is that we CAN change the level of fullness that feels normal, with practice. Our brain has something called neuroplasticity. We do grow new brain cells, and, in a nutshell, neuroplasticity debunks the old myth that you can't teach an old dog new tricks. We can reset our fullness meter by eating slower. Remember is takes about 20 minutes for leptin to set in. Eat slower and pay attention to when we feel satiated. Not full, satisfied. When we feel satiated, stop. Just stop eating, no matter how much is left on the plate. If you, like most of us humans, have a reluctance to 'waste' food, that's ok. Let me offer you a counter to your 'eating it is using it' argument. Isn't eating something you don't want or need just as much of a waste as throwing out extra food? And it's a harmful one at that! It's actually the worst option: taking on extra calories, stressing the pancreas, arteries, gaining body fat, putting pressure on the digestive system, increasing lethargy, I could go on, but you get the idea. Would you eat an old sock that's worn out, just to not waste it? I hope that's a no. No point in damaging our bodies and shortening our lives, in an attempt to not be wasteful of food. We are never going to get it exactly right when preparing/buying food. There will always be some waste. That is ok. Accept this fact. And I will add that eating extra food will not save any person anywhere else on this earth, it only serves to harm us. Good self-care would be to wrap it up for tomorrow, freeze it, compost it, give it to a friend/neighbor/pet, just don't run it through our digestive system. Digestion is hard on our bodies, especially when what we eat isn't good for us and overeating exacerbates this fact. I know how hard this can be, especially when eating with others. If they cooked the food for us, it might hurt their feelings that you didn't eat it all. Bad day at work? We deserve to 'veg' out with a pile of yummy food, right? If only it really was a 'veg' out. Also, if you're a woman eating with a man, we simply cannot match them 1:1 on food. Making our plates look just like his will mean overeating for us, unless of course he is undereating, or a smaller human than you. Lots of love is shown in this country using food and we have learned to use food to meet needs that we otherwise don't see we have. I won't go into this in this book, but I encourage you to read Mark Tyrrell's 9 emotional needs. (Perhaps a Body on Emotions book?) Let's learn what our needs are and meet them in healthy ways. If it's challenging for you to stop before your plate is empty due to other's being around, I suggest including them on your secret research project. Tell them you're experimenting with stopping eating when you feel satisfied, you want to see if you'll feel better than when you eat to fullness. Maybe they'll join you on your crazy food research project. I know we also have an innate survival instinct buried deep in our brain stem. It says to us... "hey, they are getting more than me, I might starve. Eat more, eat more, eat as much as them and one more bite." I joke, but seriously, this really happened a long time ago...those that weren't willing to fight for food would die. It's built into our DNA now, compete for food in order to survive. For this one, just knowing this is going on can stop it. If our cousin gets the last chicken leg, we are not going to starve today. I actually remember one time at my Grandma Ritter's house feeling envious that my cousin Steve ate the last bologna sandwich when I wanted it. I wasn't hungry any longer, but I wanted it anyway. I felt angry at him for eating it. So angry when he asked me if I wanted to go throw football with him, I said no. Even though I loved throwing football with him. All because he got the last bologna sandwich. In my defense, you don't have to be hungry to eat just one more bologna sandwich, right? I had no idea what was going on at the time. Now, I know it was just my survival instinct kicking in. Nothing personal to Steve, I just wanted to live, and that bologna sandwich represented living to my brain. There was no famine in the land, but my precious brain was protecting me just in case. You never know! I thought a pandemic wouldn't happen in my lifetime, and here we are. The more we practice stopping eating when satisfied the easier it gets and one day (without even noticing) we will stop when satisfied with no effort at all. Then, on the rare occasion that we do overeat, boy will we notice! It will be so uncomfortable. Miserable even. I once read in a book somewhere that fear can be conditioned without our awareness but cannot be eliminated without it. I believe our level of fullness works the same way. It can be conditioned without our awareness, especially when we're young, but it will require our awareness to change it to a new normal.

Hey, I just thought of another fun thing to do. Take just the next three evenings and cut your dinner in half. Only eat half. Then, on day 4 eat your full amount again. Eat every morsel and notice how full you feel. Tell someone about your experiment and what it felt like. Write about it in your personal research journal.

Humans can go for weeks without food with virtually no ill effects. So, don't worry about a small hunger pang on those three days if you have them – unless you didn't eat for days prior to this experiment.

Another test for you: ignore your very next hunger pang and see what happens. Do it for just one hour. Think of food you hate, if that were the only food available would you eat it right now? Focus on what you feel. Put your mind to work on something else. Then write about it in your personal research journal.

Once we've gotten food down into our stomach and our stomach has covered it with those delicious acids and enzymes, it's ready for the small intestine. But first, let's talk about a few items that can be absorbed via the stomach. And to be clear I do mean *absorbed*, not digested. Absorption allows things immediately into the bloodstream. For starters, water is absorbed. This is nice, it can help us quickly hydrate if we need to. No complaints here. Another item that can be absorbed via the stomach is simple sugars. Woah, now. What does that mean? You know that joyous feeling you get when you drink down a cold bottle of Cheerwine or Pepsi? That instant gratification? That is the feeling of simple sugars quickly being absorbed into your bloodstream. Our unevolved brain loves this. They run on sugar, our brains, it's their fuel. However, there are lots of foods that contain brain fuel and most of them are better brain fuel than simple sugars. In a pinch, it's ok, if we're about to pass out from starvation, or low blood sugar (hypoglycemia), by all means...go ahead and pump that brain full of high fructose corn syrup. I think of it of like gasoline for our vehicles. We can give it the 87 octane with additives, or the 90, the 93, the cleaner gas with no additives. In this analogy, simple sugars would be an octane of about 10. It'll keep you alive and running, albeit not well.

Another thing that can be absorbed via the stomach is alcohol. Yep, that's right.

Ooo, ooo, here's a fun experiment. Go to the liquor cabinet right now, pour a shot of something, it doesn't matter what. Call up the timer on your cell phone. Drink the shot of liquor and hit the start on the timer immediately. See how long it takes for you to feel the effect of alcohol on your brain. Tell a friend how many seconds it took (yep, I typed that correctly... SECONDS). Roughly speaking, about 20% of alcohol is absorbed in the stomach, while the other 80% will make it into the small intestine for absorption. This explains the quick and prolonged buzz we get from alcohol. It's pretty terrible for us, and yet we continue to drink it. We tend to like things that are absorbed quickly. Our brain stem was wired for quick nutrition to help our species survive. So, it makes sense we would like quick absorption. Still, we now have frontal lobes and know better and as Maya Angelou once said (paraphrasing here), do the best you can until you know better, then do better. Please, don't feel judged, I'm still working on this myself. There are a few other things that can be absorbed in the stomach, but nothing so profound that it needs to take up space in this book, so let's move on to the next phase of digestion.

The stomach delivers food to the small intestine in 'bite sized' pieces that the intestine can handle, while the gall bladder infuses the small intestine with bile through a series of little pathways called the biliary tract. Bile helps break down food further, especially fats, to help our absorption of fat-soluble vitamins (A, D, E, and K), which are critical to our health. If you remember, fat became the villain in the '70s and '80s. The "fat is the bad guy movement" was actually led by the sugar industry because someone else needed to take the fall for our declining health. It worked, for a while. We know better now, fat isn't a bad thing (We'll talk about that more in The Body on Nutrition).

The small intestine is the workhorse of digestion. This is where the rubber meets the road, where most of the nutrient absorption happens. Arguments abound about the length of our intestines. If you do an extensive search on this topic, you'll find somewhere between 20-30+ feet, with the small intestine accounting for roughly 80%. It's weird then that it's named the small intestine, but it is probably named for its diameter rather than length. We have muscles in our digestive tract that push food through. Fiber (that non-caloric nutrient) gives our digestive track something to grip on to, to help move food through. Fiber also increases food volume and causes the stomach to stretch without increasing calories and leaves us feeling fuller. In the research, fiber appears to increase leptin (the fullness hormone) and the resultant stretching of the stomach causes a reduction in ghrelin (the hunger hormone). Eat more fiber people! It's interesting how this all works together, huh?

Now that food has made its way into our small intestine it begins the process critical to life sustaining fueling. Our bodies are designed to first burn carbs, then fat, then proteins. Generally speaking, our bodies use carbs and fats for energy and proteins for growth and maintenance, although that's really too simplistic. It gets much more complicated as proteins also get used for energy, after a longer break down period so I should leave this level of explanation for the experts.

Inside the small intestine, carbs will be turned into glucose (our brain's favorite fuel) and funneled into the blood stream and travel to our liver and muscles first. We can store about 1000 calories in the liver and muscles for immediate reserve (called glycogen now that it's in storage form and living in our liver and muscles). The feeling of hunger will dissipate when we reach this 1000 calorie point. Some glucose will stay in the blood, and the rest of what we eat will go to fat stores for long-term storage. (For some reason, I imagine fat stores to look like Arvin's store in Robbins when I was kid. Containers of candy half full and just waiting to be filled with more candy.) In fact, the body will start storing fat within 4-8 hours of the start of the meal if our consumption takes us over the 1000 calorie stored mark. OOO, ooo, I know what would be super fun right now…a word problem! Let's say I went to a well-known fast-food restaurant (not calling any names or pointing any fingers here) for lunch today at 11am. I ordered a McFlurry (Oreo, of course), a bacon clubhouse crispy chicken sandwich, fries, and just 3 little mozzarella sticks (with marinara sauce). My meal totaled 2010 calories. Assuming I was 'on empty' when I arrived at this restaurant (even though that's technically impossible unless I was dead upon arrival), how many calories will I store as body fat? And how long will it be before I feel hungry again? Using our adult averages and the rough estimate of 1000, I will store the first 1000 calories as glycogen in my liver and muscles. For simplicity, we'll say that 10 calories hang around in my blood waiting and looking for immediate action (little prostitutes). This means that I will store 1000 calories as body fat. All from just one meal. At dinner time (generally 7pm for me) I'll feel hungry again because the 1000 calories in glycogen is getting low and my body does not want to use stored calories. Not unless I ignore the hunger pangs and skip dinner or participate in vigorous exercise. Only then will the body tap into my fat storage. The moral of this word problem is: If you're gonna eat a McFlurry make sure it's Oreo! Just kidding, actually the moral is: we can't stave off hunger by front-loading calories. Although I've been known to try in times where my next meal was nowhere in sight! The good news is…once the 1000 stored calories are used, the body will turn to fat burning, or another way of putting it: it will activate stored calories from fat. Hey, and don't judge yourself if your body starts storing fat in just 4 hours after eating. Look at it this way, like a Ford you were built to last! Famine and starvation will never befall you.

When we consume food, and our body starts to process the carbs our pancreas gets involved. It produces insulin to help the glucose get into the cell where it can work its magic (growth and repair). Insulin works like a key. It fits into receptors on all our cells and unlocks the cell so that the cell can receive fuel (glucose) for growing and doing all that it does to keep us healthy. Side note, I said 'all' cells, but it's not true. Our brain cells do not use insulin. Our other organs do, but our brain is designed to not need it. Again, we are wired for survival and our brain can take in glucose without the help of insulin. So, if all else fails in terms of insulin, our brain will be the last organ alive, still chowing down on any available glucose in our bloodstream. Hoping against hope. I love our persistent petulant child brains!

Unfortunately, when we eat something too high in bad carbs or just too much food period, our glucose (sugar in our blood) spikes and the pancreas does its job by over-producing insulin to meet the glucose spike. Sounds ok so far, huh? The body is just doing its job. Here's where it becomes a problem...one of two things can happen. First, maybe our pancreas is worn out from genetic factors or from having this happen too often, so it doesn't produce enough insulin to take care of the problem of too much glucose. We end up with too much glucose floating around in our system (diabetes), gunking up the arteries, you know how sticky sugar is and so it is on the inside of our arteries as well. Or second, the excess glucose problem is handled for the moment because the pancreas produced plenty of insulin, and now there is way too much insulin running around trying to open our cell receptors. Our cells know when they are full and will refuse to let in any more glucose (unlike our hangry pie holes). They quite literally shut down the receptor thereby reducing the effectiveness of the insulin. Over time, the cell receptors get tired of this happening. And similar to how a key becomes difficult to turn in a lock, the cell receptors become resistant to insulin (otherwise known as pre-diabetes).

On the flip side, when blood glucose starts to fall the body reduces insulin and we will instead start to use glycogen (glucose's storage name when it's in the liver or muscles) as fuel. Glycogen is bulky and full of water. This is why weight loss seems fast during the first days of dieting because it's mostly water that we are utilizing. As long as there is glycogen to be used no actual fat loss will occur. On a side note, here...we humans can burn all our glycogen in 2 hours when vigorously exercising or in 12 hours if not moving. It is possible to burn it all while sleeping for some, however, it restores quickly upon eating. Ideally, we eat just enough to replenish our fuel and no excess stress is placed on the pancreas or the cell receptors, and no food is stored as fat. This is where we should be focusing on not wasting food, here at what I'll call the pancreatic level, not the plate level.

The fats we eat are broken down with the help of bile (mentioned briefly earlier), produced by the liver and mediated by the gallbladder, if you still have one. In the US, some 700,000 people have it removed each year (called a cholecystectomy), please don't ask how to pronounce that. For some strange reason, it's more likely to have a cholecystectomy if you live the Southeast. I blame fleas. Seriously, I moved into a new home in 2005 and the former owners had a dog, an indoor dog. The house sat empty for a few months, just long enough to make those little boogers really hungry. On my first night there, I woke to itching around my belly button. I pulled up my shirt to peek and had lots of fleas biting me. I spent the next hour pulling them off me and dropping them in the toilet. What happened next was scary! I started throwing up and didn't stop. Even when what I was vomiting was yellow and horrible smelling, I kept vomiting. I really thought I was dying and got myself to the urgent care. It only took one retching there at the urgent care for the Doctor to say, "that's bile, we're gonna take you to the ER." And off I went. Gallbladder surgery that night about midnight and I was as good as new! Ok, the fleas bites probably didn't have anything to do with my gall-bladder problems, but I like to think of them as causal. Maybe someday I'll survey those without a gallbladder about their flea interactions. Some hypothesize that gallbladder removal is related to water quality, but I have no idea what those fleas were drinking before they bit me. So, if you have a gallbladder here's what happens when you absorb fats. When food hits the duodenum (first part of the small intestine) hormones signal the gallbladder to contract. The contractions push bile out of the gallbladder into the small intestine. As you likely know fat likes to clump together, and it would be hard to digest and absorb a big clump. Bile is what keeps this from happening. Once bile gets involved, lipases go to work breaking down the separated fat molecules into fatty acids and monoglycerides, which pass through the small intestine. They then get turned into triglycerides and combine with other neat things like cholesterol and form a chylomicron, which makes it water soluble, and it then can travel through lymph vessels and eventually into the blood stream (blah, blah, big words, blah blah). See why eating fats makes you feel full for longer? It takes a lot longer for our body to process fat (and even talk about it) and turn it into something that we can actually use. Although fat isn't the first fuel source, our body can and does use fat as a fuel source. Particularly our muscles, lungs, and heart. Think of all this like a bank account. You probably have some cash, a checking account, and a savings account, perhaps even a money market account or IRA. Refined sugars are like cash (get to it quickly), healthy carbs (turned into glycogen) are like a checking account and fat is like a savings account. Fat supplies the fuel for long duration, low to moderate movement (which our body needs/must have even – The Body on Movement). One other interesting feature of us humans is that when we start to burn body fat, (due to the fact that we've run out of our glycogen store in our liver and muscles) we will actually begin to break down our muscles first for a short period of time because body fat has no glucose in it and our brain needs fuel constantly. Greedy thing. (Isn't it kinda funny that our brain is made up of approximately 60% fat but can't use bodyfat as a fuel?) A part of the proteins (amino acids) can break down into glucose (called gluconeogenesis) so our brain can still have a fuel source. This is a short-term solution, our brain will shortly switch to burning keto-acids, which are made from burning bodyfat.

Lastly, but not least in our absorption journey is the protein we eat. Protein would be the money market account or the IRA in my earlier analogy. It's the last to be used as fuel. In fact, I've seen evidence of protein staying in my system for as long as 3 days. I have no idea if that is valid and I'm not looking it up because I can just imagine the pictures that would come up on Google if I did. And we can't unsee. Just know that proteins hang around in our body longer than carbs and fats. And again, like fat, this is why we feel satiated for longer when we eat protein. Proteins can be broken down into glucose for use as fuel, although it's still the body's third choice for source of fuel. Protein has lots of other uses too, like helping you grow and repair nails, bones, muscles, etc. They play a role in our immune system. They help carry vitamins, minerals, sugars, cholesterol, and oxygen through our blood stream and reach the cells and tissues that need them. They give tissues, muscles, and organs their shape and help them work properly. Some proteins even store nutrients (iron) so we have a backup supply. Proteins are commonly referred to as building blocks and for good reason. It's really protein's main role, but if we run out of carbs and fats, the body will turn to it to pick up the slack and create fuel. Imagine a marathoner here, who has virtually no body fat storage. They can't possibly eat enough carbs to carry them through a 26-mile jaunt. They have protein to thank for their enduring abilities to get to the finish line.

One final thing I haven't mentioned here, but feel I must, since I'm now considered a senior, ugh! Absorption takes a turn for the worse as we age. That doesn't mean we can't do things to promote it, we can. But, for this book, just know that as we age, we get worse at absorbing foods. And if you, like I, have missing organs, it's even more critical that we Absent Organ Crew (The AOC) do personal research as we age to be sure we're getting everything we need to live healthy and happy lives. Oh, and for those who are missing a gallbladder, our liver still produces bile, we're just missing our storage facility, so it heads straight for the intestine. This is why eating fatty foods can be a bit harder on us in the CC (cholecystectomy club).

The last stage of food in our body is...you guessed it. The large intestine. When we've extracted all the nutrients we need from our foods, our body pushes the leftovers into the large intestine. Did I mention that this whole squeezing and pushing process is called peristalsis? I love this word, say it. It's pronounced exactly the way it looks. It sounds so dignified, and for such a messy and smelly process. Finally, the wordsmiths got it right. Of course, I'm not considering here any of the toxin removal or the microbiome of the intestines. That's a much longer and even stinkier story for someone else to tell. I promise you there will never be a book by me named The Body on Poop.

Dr. Michael Dansinger at Tuft's University runs a weight loss clinic. He says that the main driver of weight loss is caloric reduction through dietary change. He estimates it to be 80% what you put in your body and 20% how you move your body. So, listen to and learn from your body. It is talking to you. If you give it the right 'fuel' it will run well. And remember, diesel won't run a gas engine! Just ask my dad's cousin, Johnny. Inside family joke, but for those astute out there, I'm guessing you know what Johnny did without me even having to tell you.

Thanks for reading Rae's Notes and supporting my geeky habit of reading research books and materials. Don't forget to try out all of Rae's Recipes. They are sure to make your coming days fun and entertaining with lots of great dinner time talk. And if you don't have anyone to talk to over dinner, feel free to send me your journal. I love reading, so much so, I even do it while I'm eating dinner. Email it to me at livemoorecoaching@gmail.com.

Rae's Recipes

Overuse of willpower causes fatigue. I'm living proof of that statement. After a year of no added sugars, I ate an entire cake by myself on my birthday. Shhhh! Don't wear out the self-control part of your brain. With all these recipes, try them once or however long the recipe calls for. Learn from them. If you notice something about yourself that is helpful, use that information. You are the expert on you. Not me. If your body and brain feel great all the time, keep doing what you're doing. If not, do your own personal research. Also, know that stress and anxiety will take a toll on willpower. For help with that, perhaps I could write Rae's Notes: The Body on Stress. I shamelessly recommend my own books. Not because I think they're great or the best out there. Healthy living is costly!

Recipe #1: Sneaky Snake Bites

What food you choose does not matter in this recipe. Choose whatever food you like and whatever meal is your favorite of the day. If you eat with others, don't tell anyone you're following this recipe. Be sneaky and use a timer and without changing a thing, start the timer when you take your first bite of the meal. Stop the timer when you finish your last bite. Write down how long it took to eat that meal and how you feel in your journal. Focus on physical body feelings, but feel free to add emotions as well (always). Using your same favorite meal of the day, on the following day use your timer and slow down just enough to add 5 minutes to your total eating time. Pay attention to how you feel and if you're eating with others, notice how long it takes them to eat today's meal. Write about this in your journal. What's different about how you feel after this meal as compared to yesterday's?

Journal:

____

____

____

____

____

____

____

Recipe #2: Ghrelin Hairball

If you've ever seen a hairball coughed up by a cat, you'll understand the name of this recipe. Hairballs have no food in them, so bizarre how that happens! Anyway, this recipe has no food in it, so I thought the name was appropriate. Have your timer handy and by timer, I mean cell phone. The next time you feel hunger, start the timer. Do nothing about it, just notice it. Do not eat. When your hunger subsides, note the amount of time it took in your journal, but don't stop your timer from running. Keep paying attention and note how long it takes for the hunger pang to come back. Trust me, it will. Ghrelin has never failed anyone. Write down the time. Let's go one more round, if you're up for it. Ignore that second hunger alert and note how long it is until it goes away. When you feel hunger for the third time, then you can eat whatever you want, as much as you want and as fast as you want. What did you notice about the time it took for hunger to reappear after ignoring your first and second pangs? Write down your observations in your journal. Also, write down any feelings you had while you were ignoring your hunger. Will anyone admit panic?

Journal:

____

____

Recipe #3: Leptin Slushie

Get a timer ready. When you are about to take your first bite of the meal, start the timer. Eat whatever foods you want. The food chosen doesn't matter in this recipe. What does matter is that you eat your food slowly. Chew a lot! Really, I mean make a slushie of your food before swallowing each bite. Stay totally present for the entire meal so you can stop the timer as soon as you no longer feel hunger. Really pay attention to you. There is a point in every meal where hunger turns off, listen to your body and you can feel leptin taking over your hunger controls. Write down the amount of time it took for your leptin to take over in your journal. Try this recipe over and over again. I suggest doing it a few times when you feel very hungry, and when you're just mildly hungry. Compare the times and levels of hunger you felt when starting. What did you notice? Write it down in your journal.

Journal:

____

____

____

____

____

____

____

____

____

Recipe #4: Stomach Stew

Eat anything you want for dinner over the next 4 nights.
For the first three evenings cut your dinner in half. I
literally mean, fill your plate the way you normally do and
then get half of it off your plate before you start eating.
Do NOT cheat or this recipe won't work. Eat your 'half'
meal and immediately write in your journal how that
feels. Write about it all three nights. Be honest with
yourself. If you feel cheated, write it! If you feel hungry,
write that. Or sad, or angry at me, or surprisingly
satisfied, joyful, or giddy, write it all down. Focus on how
you feel. Feelings. They have a lot to say, those little
messengers. Then, on day 4 eat your full meal again. Eat
every morsel (even if you feel satisfied before you get
done) and notice how you feel. Write that down in your
journal and compare this to the first three nights. What
differences do you notice? Also, notice differences at
bedtime and sleep quality. Write those observations in
your journal the next morning.

Journal:

____

____

____

____

____

____

____

Recipe #5: Tasty Brain Morsels

No timer needed on this one and you can eat whatever you want and as much as you want. Get foods that you are or have been craving. For one full day, eat every meal this way: start with the food you are craving the most. Eat it in its entirety. In your journal describe the taste, the texture, and what you liked about that first food item. What do you think your body was needing for you to crave this food the most? Write about your speculations in your journal and how it felt to consume it first and all at once.

Journal:

____

____

____

____

____

____

____

____

____

____

____

____

Recipe #6: Delectable Dessert

For this recipe you'll need your favorite dessert. Cake, pie, M&Ms, Little Debbie, whatever it is no matter how bad it is for your health, go get it now. Get your journal ready, you need it during this recipe. Take one bite. Just one. Chew. Pay special attention to this first bite. In your journal describe its taste, texture, what you love about it, what makes it your favorite (or top 5 if you're like me and can't settle on just one). When you're finished writing, take the second bite of it and a third. What are the differences between this bite and the first? Take a fourth bite and a fifth and let's really go for it here...polish that thing off! Be totally honest, how does the last bite compare to that first one?   Write about that in your journal. How many bites do you really think it would take to get the glorious joy of dessert, without the diminishing returns? Write that number down in your journal.

Journal:

____

____

____

____

____

____

____

____

____

Backword and Acknowledgments

The writing of this book was no monumental effort. In fact, all it really amounts to is I had free time and wanted to read what interested me, so I did. After doing so, I started taking notes and typing them. Then, after a conversation with my sister in the car on the way home from Tennessee, I pieced my notes together in a fashion that made sense to me and added in a few stream of consciousness thoughts. Oh, and on that day home from Tennessee (June 19th) my sister challenged me to finish this first short book by July 11th, when I was leaving for a week in the mountains with my new RV and a couple of buddies. My sister knows that a challenge is exactly the way to get me motivated about something and I delivered the first incredibly rough draft to her on July 9th.

Therefore, I need to acknowledge my sister for believing I could pull this together. Period. And in such short time. Your encouragement and excitement inspired me to do it. Thank you for helping me find a use for my nerdy habits and for believing in me. You are the greatest sister on earth. I'm so grateful that I got you.

Second, I'd like to thank Daffie and Tim, the world's greatest friends, for letting me use and abuse their home and Wi-Fi. Oh, and for the vodka that helped me anesthetize my stress so I could get this done.

Third, I'd like to thank Beth Knott, my co-teacher and friend who recommends a large portion of the things I read.

And lasty, Jack. For sitting quietly with me while I wrote. Even if you really were only there hoping a treat would jump off the table now and again. Shhhhh! Our little secret.

References for The Body on Food

Tara, Sylvia. *The Secret Life of Fat*. First ed., W. W. Norton & Company, 2016.

Sears, William. *Prime-Time Health*. First ed., Little, Brown and Company, 2010.

Arden, John Boghossian. *Rewire Your Brain: Think Your Way to a Better Life*. John Wiley & Sons, 2010.

Porter, William. *Diet and Fitness Explained*. Self-Published, 2021.

Bryson, Bill. *The Body: A Guide for Occupants*. Anchor Books, a Division of Penguin Random House LLC, 2019.

Lee, Kings SC. *The Five-Door Strategy to Health Weight and Happy Life*. Self-Published. 2018.

www.ingramcontent.com/pod-product-compliance
Lightning Source LLC
Chambersburg PA
CBHW051250150726
48001CB00019B/2282